T0021803

EAST MEETS WEST

Chinese Chi Healing for
Western Sexual Disorders

June Kwok

iUniverse, Inc.
Bloomington

East Meets West
Chinese Chi Healing for Western Sexual Disorders

Copyright © 2012 June Kwok

The information, ideas, and suggestions in this book are not intended
as a substitute for professional medical advice. Before following any
suggestions contained in this book, you should consult your personal
physician. Neither the author nor the publisher shall be liable or responsible
for any loss or damage allegedly arising as a consequence of your use
or application of any information or suggestions in this book.

iUniverse books may be ordered through booksellers or by contacting:

iUniverse
1663 Liberty Drive
Bloomington, IN 47403
www.iuniverse.com
1-800-Authors (1-800-288-4677)

Because of the dynamic nature of the Internet, any Web addresses or
links contained in this book may have changed since publication and
may no longer be valid. The views expressed in this work are solely those
of the author and do not necessarily reflect the views of the publisher,
and the publisher hereby disclaims any responsibility for them.

Any people depicted in stock imagery provided by Thinkstock are models,
and such images are being used for illustrative purposes only.

Certain stock imagery © Thinkstock.

ISBN: 978-1-4502-8571-1 (sc)
ISBN: 978-1-4502-8572-8 (e)

Printed in the United States of America

iUniverse rev. date: 12/28/2010

Contents

"If you've ever had questions about sexual fitness, healthy lifestyles (physical and mental) and a good, proven philosophy of life, then spend some time with June Kwok's latest book East Meets West.

"June's book has the double advantage of being grounded in her knowledge of ancient Chinese health practices, and 10 years of practical experience with thousands of clients in her Clinics located throughout Vancouver."

Good fortune, Ms Writer!

USA EDITOR

June Kwok's new book "East Meets West" is packed with valuable insights culled from her many years of experience in bringing the healing power of ancient Chinese traditions to the West. The fact that her healing skills have helped so many people is testimony to her craft.

But what arises from the pages of this book is June's deep commitment and love for her fellow man, not to mention her spritely spirit and keen sense of humor.

June's mission, as she points out in the book, is to use her vast experience to now teach others what she has discovered. "East Meets West" is an important step in that journey.

Jim Houston
Los Angeles
February 2010

Introduction & Overview

June M. Kwok is a licensed alternative health care professional providing exceptional healing therapies for a variety of conditions related to creating and maintaining excellent physical, mental, and spiritual well-being.

Clients visiting June's Pure Chi health care facilities can choose from a variety of healing modalities, including:

- Pure Chi energy practice
- Healing touch massage
- Meditation
- Chinese sacred song, sound and music
- Relaxation and breathing techniques
- Suction cup pain relief
- Stretching exercises
- Diet and nutritional applications
- Chinese herbal medicine
- Life balancing (mind, body, soul)
- Relationship counselling

These therapies help clients achieve better life-fitness and specifically improve:

- Blood flow & circulation
- Fatigue

- Insomnia
- Bodily pains
- Stress and anxiety
- Night urination
- Urinary/genital system functions
- The immune system
- Men's and women's sexual health
- Balance of mind-body-spirit
- Feelings of confidence, well-being and vigour

Clients are introduced to Pure Chi energy healing through therapeutic touch applied to the body's pressure points. The resulting bodily vibrations improves blood circulation, thereby removing toxins and other negative energy and stimulating the flow of positive Pure Chi energy throughout the body. Clients report the improved energy flow automatically clears up a condition doctors have named 'foggy brain'.

Use of light massage gloves on the healer's hands at the Clinic is standard procedure. June provides relaxing, healing music, song and voice during all treatments.

June has more than ten years' experience teaching, counselling, and practicing in these alternative health care methods. She offers her treatments in a warm, supportive, and health-enhancing environment. All clients are greeted and treated with tender loving care.

June provides her services to people of all ages. As June says, more and more Western people are discovering the alternative health benefits of Pure Chi energy, ancient

Chinese health care practices, and Reiki therapy. These do not replace Western notions of health and well-being, but compliment them instead.

Body, Mind, Soul

The interplay of 'Body, Mind, and Soul' is one of the oldest notions in many cultures. Throughout the history of Chinese culture, there have been a large number of books written on the interplay and balance of these three entities. Today, Chinese health practitioners continue to research the changing needs of humans as they balance their bodies, minds, and souls in an ever-changing and more complex world.

There is an abundance of power and energy stored in human bodies, minds, and souls. According to this belief, almost everyone has problems in maintaining balance between them. Many physicians are working hard to understand and remedy this, to restore balance between body, mind, and soul. This is a complicated undertaking, along with the subjects that come with it – Qigong (Chi), psychology, parapsychology, nutrition, sexology, and so on. June Kwok is a leader in this field, and has discovered many techniques to help restore balance in the human system.

Elements of Pure Chi

'Chi' is a traditional Chinese word that basically means 'energy' or 'life force'. This universal energy can be used to heal the body; as the body is healed, so too is the soul. Traditional Chinese medicine is based on the Taoist view of the universe in which everything is interrelated. The ancient Chinese people knew that everything in this world and in the entire universe – human beings, animals, plants, stars, mountains, oceans – is composed of energy. They labelled this energy 'Chi'.

Western science confirmed this concept when it was discovered that energy can be neither created nor destroyed; as the physicist Albert Einstein proved, even rocks, stars and the life-giving Sun itself are composed of billions of invisible particles of pure energy.

Chi practitioners believe the human body is an energy system in which the energy – the chi – moves through channels called meridians. Chi moves through the body smoothly when the body is in balance. When the movement is blocked – by physical, mental, or spiritual obstacles – the body will be in an unbalanced state – vulnerable to pain, mental distress, and disease. For optimal health, the aim is to keep Chi flowing freely through the body.

'Pure Chi' is a powerful healing therapy adapted to

Western usage by June Kwok over a period of several years while working with thousands of clients. In June's words, "Pure Chi provides food for the soul, rest for the mind, and health for the body."

Pure Chi, with its healing practices and philosophy, has endured among millions of Chinese people because it works quickly, effectively, and dependably to heal and invigorate without the use of medications or surgeries. June's healing techniques remove negative, toxic energy and blockages from your system, allowing you to experience the positive, healthful energy within you.

Chinese Sexual Arts & Men

Since ancient times, the Chinese have recognized that the body needs to have sexual balance. The body is a living thing that has needs and responses. No matter how intellectual one may be, the body requires sexual activity and touch, just as it needs good food to thrive. Sexual energy must be balanced.

In youth, men have an abundance of sexual energy, but age and overuse can dissipate this energy, and even injure performance.

The techniques of Chinese sexual arts are derived from the Tao, the Enlightened Way. These techniques train you how to use the sexual muscles surrounding the genitals for better sexual performance. Chinese sexual arts help the mind and sexual organs connect, and give a person better control over dysfunctions such as premature ejaculation or difficulty in maintaining an erection.

A trained therapist uses healing touch on various pressure points on the body to help sexual energy flow correctly. The therapist's knowledge and experience help determine the reason(s) for the person's dysfunction. The problem can be mental or physical (for example, poor performance in an aging body, or lack of control in a younger man), or a combination of the two.

Different treatments are suited to different problems. But the goal in all treatment is to use healing touch to clear blockages of toxic, negative energy; improve circulation; and exercise the affected part of the body in order to strengthen the surrounding muscles.

Ninety per cent of losing sexual energy and premature ejaculation is caused by the nerves and bloodstream being blocked by negative energy. Many people do not know how to care for the genital area of their body – how to replace sperm after ejaculation, how to allow the sexual organs to rest. Too many people simply use their body's sexual energy indiscriminately until it runs out.

Sexual energy and feeling, of course, are closely related to the health of the rest of the body, as well as the mind. Even young men can find it difficult to perform properly if they are suffering from lack of rest or exercise, insomnia, poor diet, or have been drinking too much alcohol.

Chinese sexual arts have been practiced for thousands of years because they are effective and satisfying. For a man to be in prime sexual health at any age, he first must learn self-control. This means being able to control his actions during intercourse, (e.g., the timing of his ejaculation); to control when to avoid ejaculation for the satisfaction of both himself and his partner; and also to control when not to have intercourse in order to rest and restore his sexual energy and functioning. This control involves both physical and mental techniques.

Chinese sexual arts involve techniques of breathing, foreplay, actions during lovemaking, proper hydration, rest, diet, and bodily control. These methods are very effective, but may seem unfamiliar to Westerners raised in a culture that both promotes and prohibits sexual behaviour.

For example, it is well known in Chinese culture that it can be more invigorating during sex for a man not to ejaculate, that is, not to reach orgasm while allowing the woman to do so. This requires instruction and practice, for the benefit of the man and the woman. In Western culture, strong and even multiple orgasms is a sexual goal depicted in movies and magazine articles.

It is also common knowledge in Chinese practice for the male to be able to prolong intercourse with a woman for an hour or two. This is not a rare ability performed only by an ancient sect, though it has been call Tao practice. Instead it involves a series of techniques that can be learned and applied by the man and woman sharing one another.

Men's Sexual Health

Men's sexual health encompasses physical, mental, spiritual, psychological, and emotional factors. Just as we cannot separate the mind from the body, we cannot separate a man's sexual health from all the other factors in his life. These factors include work, spouse, children, other family members, relationships with friends and business associates, diet/nutrition, physical fitness, rest, sleep, exercise, relaxation, and amount of daily stress.

The B.C. Medical Association states, "To have an erection, a whole group of things must be working right. A man's nerves and blood vessels have to respond properly, and his emotions have to aid, or at least not get in the way of, the process. Anything – physical or emotional – that gets in the way of enough blood getting and staying in the penis can cause problems with erections."

"Expectations are important, too. It is important to realize that a 35-year-old athlete is not the same athlete he was at 19, but that doesn't mean he isn't a great athlete. We don't expect him to perform the way he did 10 or 15 years ago. But, unfortunately, many a middle-aged man expects his penis to behave the way it did when he was 19. Male sexual problems have only recently begun to be talked about openly, so there has been a lack of information available to help men make better judgments about normal sexual functioning."

Additionally, as pointed out by the BCMA, "almost all men have had at least a few experiences when they wanted an erection and didn't get one, or when they lost an erection at an embarrassing point. These difficulties are common and usually temporary, and it is best to look at them as a normal part of life." (Often, an erection problem gives a man a clue about what he personally requires to enjoy good sex, i.e., a loving partner, no alcohol, good health, right location, etc.).

So, sexual health for men really means being able to perform the way he wants to sexually, taking into account various personal factors related to health and age that may cause occasional performance interruptions.

June Kwok has observed, in working with thousands of men in her Pure Chi practice, that there are some common causes – and cures – for most men's erectile problems. In the next few pages, we'll look at:

- Basic requirements for male sexual health
- Premature ejaculation
- Maintaining erections
- Loss of erectile abilities and feelings
- The age factor

With training and practice, most of June's regular clients become stronger. They find that they have more energy, are calmer, and are more at peace with themselves. In addition, they are more in control of their sexual lives. They look more energetic, they have a sparkle in the eye and their speaking voice is louder and stronger.

James, 60: Weak Erection

James appeared to be in pretty good overall physical condition when he first came to see me. However, I noticed that he had a fairly bad body odour and his hands and feet felt very cold, which indicated poor circulation, and some toxic blockage. It was autumn, with cool weather, but he was also sweating.

I asked James to lie down and tested the energy flow in his body by beginning to touch him. Touching shows me where some of his problems are. In my Chi practice, when my hands feel hot to a client, it means that area of him is cold, or suffers from poor circulation. The smell of the body or mouth also shows the state of the inner immune system.

The area around the eyes and a person's skin both can reveal the state of a person's energy. How a person talks, weakly or strongly, also is an important clue to a person's state of health. I consider all of these factors together with my experience and knowledge and I can usually guess why a person has come to me for help.

I told James that he would feel some results immediately after the first treatment, more improvement after a second treatment and, after a third visit, all should be functioning well. His body also benefited from the good genes he inherited from his family – good bone structure, well-developed muscles, and general vitality. He had been suffering from his erectile problem for only about a year, so his difficulty was easy to deal with. I explained that when I cleared up his toxic, negative energy, his blood flow and circulation would improve. Good food, fluids, rest, and some muscle exercises would strengthen him and speed his recovery.

Chinese sexual arts strengthen the body and spirit, making it more difficult for negative energy to reside there. Although often unknown to North Americans, the Chinese sexual arts help a person to hold off sexual climax longer, extend the time of sexual activity, and make a person ejaculate with quality, not quantity.

When I talked to James, he disclosed several symptoms: his sleep quality was not good, and even when he slept for 10 hours he still did not awaken feeling refreshed and energetic. He said that, emotionally and spiritually, he always felt tired. In addition, he found it hard to concentrate, his memory seemed to be getting poorer, and he got upset over little things. All of these things resulted in his erectile difficulties: he thought his penis seemed small and was losing hardness.

Sometimes he thought he ejaculated too quickly and felt that he could not control his sex life anymore. Every day he lost a little more hope, like a fading flower, until he saw my ad in a newspaper. He saw that I treated symptoms like his and came to me hoping I could do something for him. Without him telling me anything, I told him all the problems he had, and how long he had been suffering. He was shocked at my accuracy, and he started to feel calm and trust me, because I knew his body.

I gently explained to him my 15-minute rule: In practice, if he couldn't control his orgasm for 15 minutes or longer, he could be coming too early for the satisfaction of his partner. The downside of this is potentially shortened pleasure for himself.

I began to massage James to start the process of calming his body while sending pleasurable signals to him via his mind. While massaging, I questioned him further about his lifestyle. One important subject I broached was his daily water intake (urban myths abound regarding daily minimums, but I have found that many people with sexual problems drink very little water). The body, including its sexual functions, requires proper hydration. Always check with your doctor if you have a medical condition affected by water intake.

Unfortunately, James was drinking only a little water each day. I liken the body to an automobile and water to gasoline. Without enough water, physical exertion can quickly drain a person, leaving him with a physical system trying to put on the brakes in compensation.

For most people without a medical problem, as with any exercise, a drink of water should precede and follow sex. This will replace the fluids lost in this activity. I have yet to figure out an optimum method of replacing water during sex with a partner without throwing water on the activity! After ejaculation, a peaceful 20-minute rest is also very restorative.

I also showed this client some gentle stretching techniques to tone the body and calm the mind.

Because James had reached 60 and his sex life in his younger years had been very active, (four or five times a week discharge), I advised him to take it easy for one month; I told him to try not to ejaculate more than once or twice a week.

He needed to conserve his energy and sperm. When a man is young, his ejaculation is strong, but it is not the same as he gets older; that is because of the energy needed to push the sperm. This energy comes from eating protein-rich foods, getting restful sleep, and drinking enough fluids.

After two weeks, James came to see me and told me that he was already feeling better and sleeping better, and had reduced his sexual activity to twice a week. And he said his penis was twice as hard as it used to be.

John, 35: Premature Ejaculation

John had the following characteristics: premature ejaculation, allergies, problems with his nerves, very big body, and chronic shortness of breath. My first action was to give him a thorough back massage. When I had him flip over, it was evident that his nose and sinus passages were quite plugged. This was caused by breathing mostly through his nose.

I asked him to open his mouth and put his tongue behind his upper teeth. This tongue method acts as an energy connection between the mind and the penis. Energy flows from the head to the body via the tongue. I suggested that when he has sex he should try breathing through his mouth, keeping his tongue behind the upper teeth.

This would reinforce a proper breathing method and provide needed oxygen for sex. I demonstrated how to make a big inhalation until the lungs were full, then a slow exhalation. Also, I instructed him on how to breathe properly during sex and it worked. Instead of ejaculating quickly in five minutes or less, he was able to hold off for 20 minutes or more.

John was quite tense in my office at first, giving me an excellent opportunity to run him through some breathing routines to calm him down and connect his overall feelings with sexual goals. I told him to close his eyes and put his tongue behind his front teeth. In a quiet, soothing voice, I asked him to relax and walked him through a physical review of his body from head to toe.

During this process, I had him breathe in to fill his belly, then blow slowly out without moving the tongue (three times). Next, I asked him to slowly open his eyes. He felt better, more relaxed. Checking his breath, I noticed the signs of a heavy smoker. I continued coaching him through the breathing exercise for another seven repetitions. I emphasized that by using this breathing routine he could gain the physical control he was seeking during sex.

I turned on some soothing music and started singing to him gently, getting him to close his eyes and enjoy my touch. I stopped massaging after a couple of minutes and had him open his eyes because he said he was becoming too aroused. He mentioned again his problem of premature ejaculation.

So, I told him to put his tongue behind his top front teeth again and draw in a good, filling breath. I suggested that he relax and not get too sexually high. My advice was for him to feel mellow, all the while remaining aroused. Even with a naked lover in view, a relaxed attitude is beneficial. When about to come, slowing down for a couple of movements will extend the duration of activity. I told him to suck in his breathing, and use his mind to imagine the sperm running up from the testicles to inside his body. Then, for a moment or two, he should concentrate on his breathing instead of getting too aroused.

I gave John the following instructions to use when he got home: while using his hand, breathe; hold the breath until the hand is completely down to the bottom of the penile shaft before exhaling. He was told to repeat this for approximately three minutes. He found he could control his 'high' through breathing at a controlled rate.

Next, I told him to match the strokes to his breathing, but holding or only moving slightly on the exhalation. He worked up to a five-count while stroking (on the inhale), then held off while he exhaled. The goal with this routine was to train him to listen to his breathing, shutting out as much external distraction as possible.

When a man concentrates on his breathing, he can better control his level of excitement, and the body is oxygenated. An aroused body state is achieved, yet the mind is actively engaged and controlled. The result is more success and pleasure for the individual and for his partner.

Another element to keep in control is vision. If the lady in view is causing too much of a high too quickly, close the eyes for a while! But, don't concentrate too hard, to the point that you start to lose interest – open your eyes again! It is always a balancing act to control your level of excitement and sexual duration to ensure the maximum amount of sexual pleasure for you and your partner.

I suggested that he could also talk a little during sex to calm the flow of the mind, and not to concentrate wholly on his own body and penis. This, too, would save him from coming too soon. Too much centering on the sexual organs can be over-stimulating and result in premature ejaculation. By taking the break and having a drink of water, his over-revving engine can also have a chance to settle down.

Another method to delay ejaculation is to simply stop everything, withdraw from the vagina for a moment, then continue, thrusting back in. The other option suggested was to change the sexual position. It is not necessary to go into a long explanation with your partner as to why you are making the change, just flow along as part of the sex act. If you can extend the time and please both parties, then pursue it!

I asked John if he came quickly when masturbating and he said yes to that too. Quite simply, without a woman there, he was just doing it for himself and ejaculated quickly. It became apparent that this had been his practice for years. I explained that too much quick masturbation was a major cause of premature ejaculation when having sex with a partner. He had trained his sexual system to just have a quick bit of fun, and it had been transferred to sexual intercourse, even though it was not desirable.

This is how a decent fellow can unintentionally appear to be a selfish lover to his partner. In addition to the breathing techniques, I told him to learn to masturbate for 15 minutes without coming, to allow his system to get accustomed to a longer pleasure time before orgasm. Longer masturbation time conditions the individual to accept more titillation before coming. As well as concentrating on breathing and stroking, one can incorporate variations to help extend the pleasure time before orgasm. Actions such as stopping temporarily, varying the speed, opening your eyes, stopping a fantasy or changing it, all aid in keeping the mind in charge of the body. John agreed to work with these suggestions.

Tom, 55: Impotence

Tom was worried about keeping an erection and about the size of his sex organs. Sometimes a client is too mind-oriented rather than penis-centered, the result being difficulty maintaining an erection, rather than premature ejaculation. Tom had a trim body. When he lay down on the massage table at my clinic, he told me his problems with getting and maintaining an erection.

He had been feeling some shame about this as a result, and tended to avoid having sexual intercourse. I examined his body and found that he looked good, smelled good (non-toxic), and had good breathing. I asked him to tell me about his sex partner. It turned out there wasn't one. He was divorced, but he hadn't worked on finding a new partner.

He found that when he lacked a strong emotional attachment to a partner, he had difficulty getting aroused and would go soft quickly. As part of his treatment, I started to sing softly to relax him and massaged his body to make him feel good. I spoke quietly and told him that he was safe in my room, that he was handsome, healthy, and sexy.
I told him it was okay to let his feelings out and to allow himself to get aroused. I asked him to close his eyes and visualize the lady he loves or open them to visualize me as a temporary girlfriend. He opened his eyes and looked at me and his breathing started getting heavier and he said he was becoming aroused.

I continued to massage his body but, suddenly, he said he no longer felt aroused. Because of this, he felt guilty and apologetic. He didn't know what to do and displayed a marked drop in confidence. I spoke to him softly, continued his massage and told him to let himself relax. There were so many ways to help this client, but first he had to open his heart, trust himself, and want to be helped. He needed to express his feelings. While taking in my verbal lessons, he started to feel better. I kept talking to him, softly and gently.

I told him he had the best body I'd seen all day! He needed more energy, needed his mind to be opened up and not be ashamed. I asked him if his family background was of the closed-mind variety. He said it was. I asked whether his mother told him not to touch himself when he was a boy – yes again. He told me he was never accepting of his sexual organs, and that he thought he was not big enough when erect.

With a positive voice, I told him again that he had a good, strong body. It turned out that, as with so many men, he compared his own body with those in the X-rated videos. I told him not to compare himself to others. I said if he wanted somebody to like him, he first had to like himself.

I pointed out that an erection in the 4½-inch range was a good, medium size – an 'international' size. This gave him a big emotional boost. He smiled and thanked me for helping restore some of his lost sexual confidence.

Tom said that his ex-wife used to complain to him that his penis was too small. I explained to him that some women who weren't thinking correctly could be comparing a normal-sized penis with oversized sex toys or the extreme erections achieved by X-rated movie stars. However, people should not confuse size with effectiveness. I explained to him that the hardness of the penis was the important feel to a woman's vagina, and not so much the size. Basically, a really hard, shorter penis would feel much better than a longer floppy one. On the flip side, women are different too! Basically, it is the love and the feelings that count.

Many couples live with infrequent intercourse because they have loving, cuddling, close relationships. So, with a loving couple, bumps in the sexual road due to health or age are not show-stoppers. After I related this to Tom, his confidence increased somewhat. I told him that when he got home he should practice the technique I had taught him about how to pump himself whenever he started to go soft. He would then teach himself how to be able to slow down a little but keep his 'horny' edge until he wanted to 'let go'.

Michael, 50: Control Issues

I've seen Michael several times. The first time I saw him, he said he was divorced and hadn't been with a woman for four years. He was very sensual and easily excited. In order to allow him to calm down and enjoy the session, I gave him a good body rub to familiarize him with my hands, my voice and how I looked. This helped make him comfortable. He started to react. I then began to coach him on his breathing. It was apparent that he'd lost some of his confidence. He was amazed to find himself a bit out of control. I coached him back into a mind/body balance.

His problem was that he could not come without feeling love for his female partner. His expectations are high, so he finds it difficult to trust others. In the end, he always stops short of orgasm when he is with a woman, unless he has strong feelings for her. On one occasion, he could not come even after two hours of sex because of his feeling of emptiness and lack of emotion.

He said he had been with several different women over the previous two years, but that now his sexual feelings were not as strong or sensitive as they used to be. He said he could find release only by using his own hand. He told me that he used to be able to make love for hours. He didn't appear to be suffering from low energy, poor health, or emotional problems, but told me he had smoked a lot of marijuana from age 25 to 40. He said he and his wife had made love nearly every day and he was proud that he could bring his wife to orgasm several times when they had sex.

I told him his ex-wife probably now has a lot of problems with her health from overindulging in sex. He was shocked, but agreed, saying that she now cannot work and has a lot of problems related to hormone irregularities. He said her doctor has advised her that her immune system is not strong and she has poor blood circulation. He no longer finds her attractive and says he feels sorry for her.

I explained that the body is a bit like an engine, and when you overwork it sexually, it wears down over time. From age 20 to 40, you may not feel any problems, but you actually use up your 'mileage', or the natural body energy that you inherited genetically from your parents.

Even if you inherited good health and a strong body, these can be abused by over-use. Other not-so-lucky people may be born with poor health because of their genetic inheritance, or because their parents drank alcohol, took drugs, or were getting too old when they conceived. This difference in parental background explains why some children's health is not as good as that of others. Parents who are young, in good health, and possessing a lot of life-energy will generally pass that on to their children.

Even with the best of health, a man's hormone levels begin to drop after age 45 (the so-called 'male menopause'). When this is compounded by the stress from an unhappy marriage, and other life stresses, it is natural that a man will feel the effects in his sexual life, too.

I told Michael that if he lowered his expectations a bit and didn't seek perfection in a female partner, his heart could still become engaged with a woman and they could enjoy one another. So, he should not get locked into being a dreamer who forgets to live life as it is.

I reminded him that it is not always easy to live with another person and that sometimes people have to be prepared to make some changes in themselves in order to be happy in a relationship. It is necessary to be able to forgive and to work out where the problems are if you want to be able to look back on your life as a happy one. It is easy to fall in love, but few couples have learned to be happy over the long term.

I told Michael that I hoped he would win a new love and

wished him good luck. He looked at me, and said he was pleased with the answers I had given him.

Now Michael is one of my best clients. Through his visits, he has managed to maintain his confidence and keep balance between his mind and body. He comes for the relaxation massages and enjoys the results, leaving happy and relaxed. Michael realizes that he still wants a good, long-term relationship and is willing to seek it. He feels he is keeping his mind and body in good shape for the lady that he will meet in future.

Mr. Johnson: The Sexy Senior

Mr. Johnson is an older man, a widower, and a good client, coming for massage to help him feel more vigorous. Like 70 per cent of men, he wants something extra besides his loving wife. He likes touch, both giving and receiving it. He is a very sensual gentleman. At home, when his wife was alive, he was a good husband and father. He wanted to be a man of quality, making his wife feel important, while keeping the spice in his relationship.

He loved his wife, but his wife was not a good lover. So, for the sake of his mind and his body, he kept his sexual feelings balanced through massage. He told me that's how he kept his marriage happy. However, two years ago, his wife died and now he is in his 70s. At that time, his health became very poor due to some surgery and medications that affected his sex life, although his sex drive was still there.

He had good memories about the sex he used to have and when he found that he could no longer react, he felt upset and disappointed. After he met a younger girlfriend, he wanted to restore his vitality. Nowadays, according to some experts on erectile dysfunction, nearly all men suffer from erectile problems at some point in their lives. Of these cases, 70 per cent are moderate and about 30 per cent are severe due to age or other conditions. Mr. Johnson falls into the latter group.

When he was younger and in the army, he damaged the function of his sex organs because he engaged in too much sexual activity each night. He was proud of his capacity, but he was a hungry wolf all the time. He said he would have sex whenever he could during his army days and would come 4 to 7 times per night when he had the chance with a lady. Next day, he said he sometimes had difficulty walking!

One day during his army life, he found he could not control his urination. This was due to having too much sex. Following a doctor's advice, he realized he needed to slow down his sex life. But the damage was already making him urinate a lot at night. This can also happen to men who are age 40-plus and have young girlfriends who they try to keep up with.

Mr. Johnson hoped to get his sexual feelings going again, which is why he came to see me. He said his sexual organs and feelings had become 'hopeless'. He found that whenever he discharged, there was little feeling. Every day he told himself, "I'm old. I just have to be satisfied that I can come."

And he continued to suffer from frequent night urination. His testicles were too weak and he needed the Chinese exercise techniques I described to him.

About three months after he saw me, he reported that he was feeling much better. Trips to the bathroom had been reduced to once a night. He saw his sexual organs come bouncing back to life and said to me, "June, you're my China doll. You saved me!"

David Meets June

David Rogers, a 31-year-old legal researcher, has finally worked up the courage to do something about a sexual problem that has been making him depressed. His wife, Susan, has been telling him lately that when they are in bed together he is not thinking enough of her needs. David is baffled by his wife's complaints because he loves her deeply and believed he was satisfying her sexually.

It turns out that Susan has always been concerned about how quick their love-making sessions begin and end, but has only recently started telling him. Because of her dissatisfaction, and his plummeting self-confidence, they have not been intimate for almost four months.

David's problem is technically called premature ejaculation, or inability to avoid ejaculation during sexual intercourse. Despite the availability of sexual information in books, on Web sites and in the media today, men often don't know how to deal with this problem.

"A lot of premature ejaculation is caused by nobody telling men what to do or how to do it, and they might not know how to truly relax sexually," says June.

"I talk with men about how to make their love-making

last longer. Whether they're with their sexual partner or looking at books, they find they cannot correct the problem by themselves."

"They are suffering, they are frustrated, and they begin to lose confidence in their sex life. After their partners complain, they start to feel lost and scared of being close to a woman. Then they refuse to listen to feedback about their sexual performance."

June deals with several male sexual problems, including the inability to get or maintain an erection, premature ejaculation, insomnia, stress, night urination, and poor circulation. All of these symptoms are related in that they can have psychological, emotional and physical dimensions, and all can affect men's sexual performance. A man who is worrying about premature ejaculation may lie awake at night and not get enough sleep. This merely adds to the problem!

June begins her therapy sessions by asking about her client's lifestyle and often finds he is overstressed and overworked. She advises clients to make sure they take time each day to eat properly, get sufficient sleep, avoid anger and stress, exercise and take time for relaxation. She also advises clients to make sure they drink enough liquids each day to keep properly hydrated, unless their doctor has advised otherwise.

Today, David finds himself at June's Pure Chi Clinic, lying naked on a padded table with a white towel draped over his buttocks. When he arrived, he was told to shower in an adjacent room and to drink some bottled water.

"David was quite tense in my office," says June. "Since it was his first visit, he no doubt had little idea as to what will happen here."

Here is some of what June shared with David:

Most people don't have any idea how wonderful it is to have true love. While you are making love with someone you truly love, your hormones are flowing, your energy is flowing, and this makes your feelings last longer and be more fulfilling. Your body, mind, and soul are nourished. This is what it means to 'make love' as opposed to just 'having sex'. There are many people who are looking for true love. They feel empty without it.

In Chinese philosophy we acknowledge that one-third of our lives is spent sleeping, another one-third is spent working or studying, and another one-third we spend serving in some way – we have countless errands, family commitments, and then we have to find time to be alone and relax. Finding balance can be so difficult.

According to recent research, about 70% of North Americans live just day to day without anything significant happening. They don't seem to care about anything. Sometimes they are suffering with making a living, they eat when they need to eat, they have sex when they need sex, they sleep and wake, they talk to their spouses and children, but they never think about how to better their souls. They just go from one mundane thing to the next and follow their typical lacklustre routine. People come to me and say that if they'd known life would be like this, they would have had more fun when they were young.

Most men nowadays have 'too much fun' when they're young, and this quickly changes when they are married with children. It seems to be one extreme, and then another. They overwork their bodies sexually at a too-young age, and by the time they're in their 40s or 50s, they've almost completely lost their sexual vitality. They've lost their libido, and consequently their zest for life.

Nowadays a lot of people start to masturbate regularly at the age of 13, especially men, and because they're not fully grown or sexually mature (their nervous systems are not yet fully developed, and their nerves in the genital region not fully grown), their sexual vitality is depleted too quickly. In this sense, they are abusing their own bodies!

Another problem is in the way masturbation is treated in many households. Children are taught that masturbation is wrong or dirty, and so when they are teenagers they masturbate in secret, and as quickly as possible so no one sees. In males, this is one of the root causes of premature ejaculation.

When these teenage males reach adulthood, satisfying women sexually becomes excruciatingly difficult because they are used to coming quickly. Sex becomes a chore, and men begin to feel great shame. Their penis is not able to stand up for two hours, let's say, and they become frustrated. They start to feel like failures in bed.

It's best to wait until you are 'sexually ripe' to begin coming regularly. Have sex instead of mindlessly masturbating. Or if you masturbate, do so with great care. You need the yin to your yang. You are the male energy, and you need the female energy to have balance. With masturbation, there is constant giving, but not getting. There is coming, but nothing to receive it. And if you masturbate too early, you greatly influence your future sexual health. But we don't think about this when we're young; we often don't find out until it's too late.

We start losing our hair, our eyes don't work as good, our teeth are not as strong. Our children grow and don't need us anymore. Family members start dying, and our hearts begin to feel like ice. We start to ask ourselves, "Is this my life? Is my life really like this? Am I going to just live this way and then die, too?" All these big questions start coming to us and we start facing different truths, possibly very negative ones. Our friends are facing health problems, because nobody has perfect health.

If everybody could live to be 200 years of age we would all be a huge success, because we learn as we get older. We start to realize the truth. We start to truly understand what we want and that life is something you can never predict; you never know how long you'll live – you could die today or tomorrow. Everything that happens to us is meant to be – you *can* change the mountain, but you *cannot* change a person's soul.

People are shaped by their environments, it's true. There are good people who become bad, just as there are bad people who become good. Environment, karma, and the people in our lives can determine the direction our paths will take.

The Chinese people have been around for thousands and thousands of years. Chinese people tend to look younger and their food is known to be the best, and the variety of the cooking, the art of cooking, is incredible. The Chinese tradition can be likened to a wise old man who has experienced a lot, has lived through so much, has learned the hard way, and can now teach others what he has found.

I moved to the West when I was 16, but I was raised in a strict Chinese home. I couldn't go out with boys – no dating, only school, homework and staying close to my family. When I moved here, I was scared to 'join the party', so I got married to the first man I dated. Then I started meeting people who had never married and they had so many sexual partners during their young lives. Some of the Westerners I met had had so many partners they couldn't even remember all of their names!

Generally speaking, these people start wanting to settle down when they're in their 30s. They want a house and a family. But they tell me that their sex lives are dull in comparison to what they had when they were younger. They miss the excitement and the many different sexual partners. There was one young man I spoke with who didn't have enough money to buy good clothes. He spent all of his energy on sex – sexual thoughts and sexual gratification – instead of on his career and bettering himself. He told me that he always thinks about sex and he wants to have fun while his body is young and still functioning properly. He becomes aroused so easily, in the morning, at night, and whenever he touches or sees an attractive woman. All of his energy is being lost to this.

So, two extremes seem to exist in Western culture regarding male sexual health: men who have too much sexual energy and men who don't have enough.

In traditional Chinese medical books, for treating erectile dysfunctions, it tells you not to come for three months. During this time give your penis a lot of rest, eat good food and herbs, exercise, and try not to get turned on. Don't hang around friends who are very sexual. You need at least three months to restore or balance your sexual energy.

I like to describe the body's energy using the image of a water hose (I'm particularly thinking of the male body!). With a lot of energy, you are able to shoot far. Without that pressure, the water runs dry, or it just falls out. We need energy to make the blood flow and to clear all the toxins that build up in our bodies.

The body listens to the mind, the mind listens to the soul, and the soul is energy. If you don't pay attention to the body's signs, the body will continue to become run down. If there is a particular problem in the soul, a coinciding part of the body is usually affected. The affected part of the body does not receive enough blood flow, and the energy becomes negative, foggy, and cold. You go to the doctor and the doctor might send you for blood tests. But the blood tests cannot test your energy, they cannot test the state of your soul. Blood tests only work when you are already damaged, when you are already sick.

The mind is the soul's office. The body is the mind's car, and the mind is the driver of the body. The body needs to function at its best, and the mind needs to be uncluttered; otherwise the soul's energy is obstructed.

Pure Chi MASSAGE

"The soul is spiritual, the mind is sensual, and the body is sexual. I find that most men in this day and age are suffering with their sexual health. I use Sexual Fitness Control to advise them in achieving better control, how to do special strengthening exercises, how to have better reactions, when to touch, how to touch, where to touch..."

—June

Senior Man I

The senior body is usually very, very sensitive. They love to touch, and they can come easily sometimes. To prevent this during the massage, a condom can be used, which can prevent being too sensitive to the touch. Just tell him how to make himself calm.

Tell him to calm down. When he's calm, put the energy to his body, his genital area. Tell him how to breathe; he needs a lot of oxygen. The body will calm. That's how I work with pressure points. Make sure he's got enough blood flow. Start a nice touch. Once the pressure point is stimulated, the blood will flow directly to the area.

Now is the time to massage him, slowly. Remind him to breathe. With the massage, I use my energy of chi, vibrating the genital area. This technique will make the client feel sensual, but not too sexual. Just by stretching, pulling, you can help strengthen muscles that can prevent excessive night urination. You can also see that some genital work will get blood flowing in the area, and the chi will clear out the toxins. Make sure the person is not over-excited by your massage technique.

Now hum, while breathing, and then focus. Focus on breathing, massage and tracking. Tell him to tighten his bum. Tell him how to hold and breathe. Pump and hold, pump and hold. Tell him to do this exercise every day when he wakes up. If you practice a good stretching exercise, a lot of toxins cannot stay in the area. The toxins, the cold air cannot stay. With a little bit of oil, tell him to pump slowly.

Still feel hope for his age; he needs new hope to feel that he's still young because his sexual organs are still alive. If my organs do not feel alive, I don't want to live. This is what a lot of men tell me. My massage work is very artistic, very spiritual. It's not easy to work on. Many men are concerned.

Sometimes testicle work is called for; this is for night urination. If it's a good massage, it will give heat to this area. With this energy, from the top to the bottom, from the outside to the inside, it can prevent night urination and may provide comfort for prostate problems. Rub, hold, then repeat the technique, following the way he feels. Make sure it's what he wants and that he's not over-excited. Ask him to rest if he needs to. Give him positive feedback, making him feel alive, making him feel oneness – the energy flows – like a circle.

Transfer your thoughts, care, love and energy to him. Stimulate him; make him feel he's in good hands. Repeating the technique, make him feel he's in heaven. The time goes fast. His entire genital area will be warmer. He's alive now, he's OK now.

If his body feels too dry, use massage oil. Massage, squeeze, touch and make him feel the flow of energy. Make him feel like he's in heaven. This is the most sensitive spot. You need to talk to him, ask him to breathe, not to get over-excited. A lot of oxygen through "the valley", that's how he'll enjoy the treatment. Slow him down through breathing instructions. Ask him to rest. And then, play nice soft music, Let him slip into peacefulness, calmness, rest.

One last massage for him again. It's time to close it up, and relax. He experiences a long-lasting sensation and he saves energy. Ask him to perform these exercises himself daily if he can, while he's standing or sitting. This will make him feel strong.

Younger Man

The younger man usually has a nice, physically fit body to work on. Massage will keep the younger man feeling fit and relaxed, and may prevent night urination from becoming a problem. Protect yourself while you're young, and then you will know that you will get better reactions for many years to come. You will know you'll have a good sex life, because you will not get overly sensitive from touching. With massaging, stimulating the pressure points, the body will automatically react.

The most sexual part of the body, I will say, are the sexual organs. This is one reason I like to concentrate on this area. It will reveal how the man feels – Is he healthy? Sick? Weak? Or is he all excited, or does he need to be touched? I teach different techniques depending on what state he is in. Locating pressure points, slowly stimulate the genital area. The person might fall asleep, depending on what mood he's in. With this massage, your mind goes nowhere. After a good massage, the genital area is very relaxed. It doesn't feel sensitive anymore.

Let the whole body relax, touching the whole body, not only the genital area. All the concentration is on the exercise, combined with breathing.

If he gets too aroused, use your other hand to touch another part of his body. Get his attention on something else. Then start over again. His feeling with be like the stock exchange – up and down! I always tell men to respect and take care of this part of their body. I think it is one of the most spiritual parts. It is connected directly the brain, the mind. A lot of what we feel comes from this area, just as what we feel effects it.

Push the pressure points, stop him from feeling he has to come, then he can save energy. Make him ease his mind and not think of coming. Just make him feel heat, warmth, and relaxation from the massage. With a healing voice, with a soft and steady touch, focus on the whole body, slowing him down, let any of his sexual feelings from the massage slowly disappear.

Senior Man II

Teach him how to exercise the genital area without getting over-excited. Ask him to focus and relax. Ask him to try breathing exercises during the massage. And like always, work with the whole body. Don't do it anymore if he gets tired.

Train him to use the muscles in his genital area while concentrating on breathing steadily the entire time. He needs to bring in a lot of oxygen. Sexual ability is just like an engine. It has a certain mileage. And at his age, for sure, there are a lot of things that he already doesn't have as much of – and energy is one of them.

Be sure to be gentle and slow. If you notice that he's very tired, ask him to rest. When he's exhausted, the quality will not be good later. Take it easy, take time, ask him to relax, the stimulate the pressure points. Make sure the blood is flowing to more than just the genital area. The blood can flow to the legs and feet as well. Stimulate one upper pressure point, and one lower, and then he can feel good and relaxed. Rub the groin and thigh area, as this will help with night urination and will clear the area of toxins and aid blood flow.

Overweight Man

Sometimes he finds himself not able to get hard enough. For sure, the massage itself will help him, but a lot of times, it's because the weight blocks the energy from flowing. So what I do is ask him to lie down and relax for a few minutes. Then, start to make him feel open. Open up his mind and the sexual channel. And then during the massage, go by his feeling. Train him to do the exercises himself, and see how much muscle he has around the genital area.

Usually it is harder to work on someone who is heavier, and it takes longer, but with the massage usually they lose weight quickly because the toxins come out of the body and the circulation gets better. The massage helps achieve overall balance.

When I am showing someone a massage technique I want my client to know that I'm truly caring for him. I don't want to make him feel sexual. I make him feel like I'm his nurse, therapist, doctor and friend. I ask him to look at himself and see how his body is working. Many overweight men are not able to see themselves very well, they can only feel.

A lot of times, overweight men don't feel as strong as the thinner guys because the body is heavy and therefore the sensations are not as strong. So I always like people to help themselves and understand that losing some weight is very beneficial for making love. A good lover is usually a thinner guy. With a heavy body, the blood doesn't flow as well. The internal organs are not as sensitive either. The heavy weight makes his breathing too heavy. The body seems to always need more oxygen. The body needs so much oxygen; it will make the body feel that the sexual organs cannot be controlled very well. That's why it's important to ask him to breathe properly and rest.

Usually overweight people cannot be rushed. A lot of healing and rest is needed for the whole body. When they are fully filled with oxygen, breathing through the mouth, not from the nose, so the body is absorbing a lot of air, that's when the genitals feel better. While massaging, it's important to notice the energy and temperature. Usually heavy people's stomachs are cold and they are not very easy to work on. If they have cold air around the area, use energy to create a nice, warm massage, from head to toe. His blood flow will quicken and energy will flow internally.

Be sure to tell him what is happening. Massage the entire genital area over and over again. Tell him what to do and what to focus on. The position is very important.

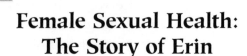

Female Sexual Health:
The Story of Erin

The atmosphere is damp and chilly as a young woman wearing a black jogging suit is running in a suburban neighbourhood. Even though the sky is clear with a few clouds hovering over, Erin begins to breathe heavily, which is a sign of low temperature. If you had met Erin two months ago, you probably would not have recognized her; especially since the drastic change in her energy levels...

Although Erin just turned 22, she had always felt tired and weak. She had suffered from insomnia for more than half a year. Even with the assistance of medication, she still had not been able to sleep well. When she was able to sleep for a long period of time, her body never felt rested. She always seemed to have colds and mental fatigue. With fading memory, she would get upset over trivial matters, like not being able to remember where she put her house keys. Erin felt something was missing. She tried to ignore her concerns at first, but continued to carry this burden subconsciously.

Since her teenage years, she had been experiencing yeast infections and irregular periods. When she was a student, she missed school several times because of severe menstrual pain. Her family doctor prescribed birth control pills to regulate her cycle, though the pain did not disappear and Erin began to engage in sexual activities. She did not realize her body was not completely mature yet, and her sexual muscles became stretched and worn out. Many young women are pressured into having sex, sometimes quite often. If a woman has sex too often, her sexual energy can be depleted by the age of 40, along with an overall decrease in vitality.

Although Erin has a care-free nature and does not cave into peer pressure, she does tend to accept romantic and sexual gestures from men. For instance, she had met a man through her roommate, who happened to be the best friend of her roommate's boyfriend. He often came over to the girls' house to hang out. He caught Erin's eye with his witty charm and sweetness. She began to feel exhausted over time, as three months went by in their relationship. He played a critical role in her physical state by not being supportive, and his sarcastic comments damaged Erin's self-esteem. He thought she was just being lazy. She initiated the break-up, yet she still had to deal with seeing him almost every day. The atmosphere around the house began to change too when she overheard her roommate, the boyfriend and her ex talking about her behind her back.

Erin hid inside her bedroom in her basement suite most of the time, but shadows of betrayal and anger followed her. Without any windows or light, her mind played tricks on her. After several months of isolating herself from social situations, a phone call from her brother, Keith, saved her. He recommended that she see a Chi therapist. Erin had always been fascinated with Asian culture since she is half Chinese. Her most memorable trip was to China, where she visited the Great Wall and the Temple of Sholin. She decided to book an appointment with June right away.

When Erin meets June for the first time, an immediate result occurs while June is performing Pure Chi Massage over Erin's head. "Although Western medicine holds that sickness is solely caused by invasive elements such as bacteria, viruses, parasites, and injury, negative energy within the body can actually cause energy blockage, forming a weakened immune system and illness." Listening to June's explanation, Erin wonders about the source of negative energy.

"When a place has been empty of human energy for a long time or is dim, that place can feel cold, or can produce other discomforts, such as recurring headaches." The image of a window with closed curtains floats across Erin's mind. "Other places may contain negative energy left behind by negative people. Sometimes we can sense this, and if we remain near this person for an hour or two, our skin absorbs the negative energy. Then we might feel dizzy or lose control of our temper easily."

"Negative people can pollute you if you sleep in the same bed, work together, or are close in any other physical way. This is similar to when you are near a person who has the flu and you are sitting in a closed space with them: you will get sick if your immune system is not strong enough." Erin let out a gasp, because this sounded uncannily familiar. "To give another example, when people enter a bar filled with smoke and leave an hour later, they are covered from head to toe with that smoky smell. The only difference is that negative energy does not give off a warning smell like smoke does. The smoke analogy illustrates how easy it is for us to soak in negative energy from the air, the environment, other people, and sometimes even ourselves. We can create negative energy when we complain or get down on ourselves constantly. This negative energy outweighs the good energy, thus affecting judgment, and that is when we need to recharge." Erin takes a moment or two to absorb the information. She sees how this applies to her experiences.

"Just as you do not drive as well on a foggy day, your mind and body do not function as well when you feel 'foggy'. You can own a very good car, like a Mercedes, but if the driver is not good, the car will not be saved from being damaged. Similarly, a good body with a weakened soul will not remain healthy for long." June hands a DVD to Erin and says, "This is my Pure Chi Meditation DVD. Ten lessons with me will help tremendously with your present condition." Erin feels determined and agrees to June's proposal.

"Drink warm liquids and eat spicy herbs; this is especially significant whenever visiting jails, hospitals, or funeral homes. Not only do you have to wash your hands, but also take a hot shower for cleansing your aura. The body craves warmth to function optimally, yet most Canadians have the habit of drinking refrigerated drinks or tap water. A cold drink of water, even on a hot summer's day, is a distinctive Western habit, not a Chinese one. Have you ever noticed that the Chinese always serve tea?" asks June. Erin nods her head in surprise because she often drinks a lot of pop and other cold drinks. "You should eat more niacin-rich (vitamin B3) food, including eggs, nutritional yeast, avocados and dried figs to open up arteries for better blood circulation. Vitamin E is known to oxygenate the blood. Vitamin E can be found in unrefined cold-pressed vegetable oils, nuts, sweet potatoes and leafy vegetables. Consuming garlic, onion, ginger, pepper, chilli, curry, and vinegar can build up your immune system and maintain your youthful appearance. You need it!" exclaimed June.

Erin then describes her period pattern and persistent yeast infections. She is frustrated with what Western medicine usually prescribes. "There are many factors that contribute to the cause of yeast infections," explains June. "The two most common ones are improper hygiene and masturbation with unclean hands. Wearing unclean or over-washed underwear, as well as frequently wearing nylons, can affect the circulation in the genital area, leading to an overgrowth of yeast. Concerning menstruation, an irritating and fatiguing period that lasts from one week to 10 days is considered irregular. Drugs prescribed by medical experts may relieve menstrual symptoms but can cause negative changes in hormones. To relieve menstrual symptoms naturally, a girl must take care of her body by monitoring eating habits carefully and drinking a product like Tahitian Noni Juice for smoother blood circulation. Replenish often with vitamins, grapes, apples, bananas, watermelon, squash, and herbs like ginseng. Cold drinks, alcohol, and raw salad including mushroom should be avoided." June sympathizes with Erin and many other young women who have these problems well into adulthood.

June shows Erin correct stretching techniques to help strengthen her genital area, and improve circulation. Stretching should be a gentle maneuver. When stretching, breathe slowly while picturing your body in a relaxed state. Listen to your inner voice. By doing regular Chi stretching for the back, you are less likely to pinch nerves and connective tissues when being sexually active, not to mention your other day-to-day activities. By stretching before sleeping and upon waking up, the muscles and joints are loosened. This improves blood circulation and one's body will be ready for new challenges ahead.

A connection has already grown between Erin and June. Besides admiring June's knowledge and skills, Erin has developed a keen interest in Pure Chi and is interested in possibly becoming one of June's apprentices.

A Married Couple's
Loss of Sex Drive

Mrs. B.: Hi, June. I would like to know about my lack of sexual feelings and what is causing this. I work quite a bit and feel tense and stressed much of the time. I feel tired and lack energy. We are both 33 years old and my husband and I would like to start a family, as we have been happily married for 8 years. We both have a low sex drive and most of the time we feel too tired to make love. What causes this lack of sexual feelings or low sex drive? My husband and I are still young.

June: Sexual feelings come from an activity centre in the brain. There is a sexual channel that is like a wire running to this part of the brain. In some cases when you feel tired, there is poor blood circulation in the brain, or lack of oxygen, and your mind begins to feel slow or foggy. Toxins are blocking the energy flow through the channel. Therefore, there is no sexual urge. Sometimes this is due to stress, tension, hormone irregularities, or other health problems. In the first years of a relationship you may be making love quite regularly, for example, four to five times a week. This may be normal when you are young but things change as you get older. As the years go by the body begins to slow or cool down and doesn't function as it did before. Some of the reasons for this are heavy work, stress, and being with the same partner. Also, energy that is lost through frequent orgasms is not being replaced quickly enough. Another common reason is that one partner may burn out or not feel as sexual, especially women after they have had children. After about 5 years of making love with the same person, in the same positions, in the same environment and the same energy, sex begins to feel more like homework. This is okay.

Mrs. B.: Is there a magic button or something we can press to turn sex drive on? I'm just kidding! I know it's not that easy, but seriously, what can people do? My husband and I would like to make love more often, especially now that we want to start a family.

June: You may have to change partners. This will excite the brain and body. However, you can do things differently to change the energy. Celebrate on special days by making love, change the environment, and try different positions. Experiment and get creative. Create a signal to let your partner know you are in the mood. If your husband is feeling sexual that day he can drink out of a certain coffee cup as a signal to let you know. Then you have all day to prepare. Just think, "tonight is the night." This can be used as a mental warm-up to help prepare your mind and body. Women usually have strong sexual feelings right before and after their period. Let your partner know this is a good time.

Sleep in separate beds or use separate blankets because when you sleep together the energy transfers between both parties. If one is unhealthy the other can begin to feel the same. Do not sleep with your pets either. Animals have different energy than humans. They have a shorter life, faster heartbeat, and a lot of toxins that can be transferred to you. You can dispel the toxic energy in the brain by doing regular Chi practice and soon you will find your sexual feelings awakening.

Mrs. B.: What can we do to make sex more enjoyable and to sustain the energy so we feel like making love more often?

June: You can prepare by eating better for a few days before sex. Eat meat and fish to increase sexual energy. Also, drink a little wine to help you both relax and drink warm water during or after sex. This replaces lost fluids and helps the energy to flow so you won't dry out, feel tired, heavy or get a headache. After sweating while your body is warm, drinking cold water is not good for the system.

If you must have oral sex, try not to orgasm at this time. Hold back, ask your partner to slow down and then proceed to have regular intercourse, and then orgasm. It is better to transfer energy through the sexual organs instead of orally. People may lose energy because there is not an equal exchange between the partners. It is also best if you can orgasm together at the same time. Use a signal to tell your partner when you are ready.

Lastly, create a routine for making love regularly, once or twice a week. Having one orgasm with a big discharge or two smaller ones will vibrate the inner system and train your system to have sexual feelings on a regular basis.

A Note from June About Karma & The Next Life

I believe a person's body dies, but the soul never dies. What you give in life, you will get back in the next. From each person (soul) that you help or hurt, you will experience the consequences – positive or negative. This explains why people are drawn to each other. This is why they either love or fight. When someone dies, they go on to be reborn in a new life, and in this new form they will get back whatever it is they gave. I don't know of any person without pain or problems – without some karmic negativity. Only your wisdom can fix these problems and end this continual karmic cycle. Know that your wisdom comes from past lives, and your wisdom can help heal you. You have been greatly challenged by your problems and you will likely have many more ahead of you, but rest assured that you can achieve peace of mind even now.

Today, I will send my dear father's soul to a better place, and I am 100% certain that my father will go to this better place. Not everyone will agree with the choices I've made in my life, but I know what my mission is and the rest I leave to God. I have lost everything in my life, including my family, and now I've also lost my father. I know, however, that I'll be very lucky in my next life, I will give back what I owe to others, and I will work my way up to higher spiritual levels. I may have to be reborn many times, but I'm not worried because I have met so many great people along the way. My heart and soul are thankful. Each day I am so thankful!

The Soul

My beliefs give me comfort, since death is just like changing homes. The soul moves from one body, one home, to the next.

The soul left this body because its time is up and it needs to depart.

The soul will carry what you owe and what your body did to others.

The soul will 'upgrade' or 'downgrade' depending on this life.

The soul cannot carry anything for you, only love and hatred.

The soul cannot be changed, except through practice and experience.

The soul needs good deeds to be strong and filled with blessings.

The soul needs prayer to connect with your inner self.

The soul you cannot see; only close your eyes to feel it alive inside you.

The soul you can hear when your heart is peaceful and calm.

The soul does not die; it only moves 'up' or 'down'.

The soul will be happy only if you follow what is right in your heart.

40 Expressions of
Wisdom for Your Life

1. Walk for 10-30 minutes every day, and smile.
2. Sit quietly for at least 10 minutes every day, preferably alone.
3. Upon rising in the morning, say "My goal for today is…"
4. Listen to quality music every day. This is real nourishment for the soul.
5. Live with the 3 E's: Energy, Enthusiasm, Empathy.
6. Play more games than last year.
7. Read more books than last year.
8. Look at the sky at least once a day, appreciating the majesty of the world that surrounds you.
9. Dream more, while awake.
10. Eat more foods that come from trees and plants. Eat less manufactured foods.
11. Eat berries and nuts. Drink green tea, plenty of water, and perhaps a glass of wine each day; toasting something beautiful in life and, if possible, in the company of a loved one.
12. Try to make at least 3 people laugh every day.
13. Don't spend your precious time immersed in rumours, things from the past, negative thoughts, or things beyond your control. It is better to invest your energy in the present.
14. Life is a school, and we are students. Problems

are lessons that come and go; what we learn from them will serve us for the rest of our lives (and maybe even longer).

15. Eat breakfast like a king, lunch like a prince, and dinner like a beggar.
16. Eliminate clutter in the home, car, and office. Let a new energy enter your life.
17. Smile and laugh more often.
18. Do not let an opportunity pass to hug a friend.
19. Life is too short to waste time hating someone.
20. Don't take yourself so seriously. Nobody else does.
21. It is not necessary to win every argument. One must accept that the other person is not in agreement, and learn from his/her position. Try to listen.
22. Make peace with your past, so as not to ruin your present.
23. Don't compare your life to the lives of others. You have no idea of the highways they have travelled.
24. Nobody is responsible for your happiness, except yourself.
25. Remember well that we have no control over what happens to us, but we do have control over how we react.
26. Learn something new every day.
27. What others think of us is not entirely under our control. Let them think what they will.
28. Appreciate your body and its marvels.
29. Whether the situation is good or bad, it will change.
30. Work will not take care of us when we are sick. Our friends will. Stay in contact with them.

31. Reject everything that is not useful, amusing, or beautiful.
32. Don't lose time. We already have all the things we need.
33. The best is yet to come.
34. Nothing is as important as sitting, standing, getting dressed, and helping others.
35. Have fantastic sex, always in harmony with the other person.
36. Phone your family regularly, and tell them, "Hi, I was thinking of you."
37. Each day, before going to sleep, say: "I am thankful for…. Today I succeeded in…."
38. Remember that we have too much that is good to be stressed.
39. Enjoy the voyage. There is only one chance to be successful.
40. Life is beautiful. Appreciate it, and be thankful.

…Have a wonderful journey, my friend!

When You Can't Sleep

It is good to stay off the Internet before bed.

It is good to have a cup of hot milk or some other liquid.

It is good to meditate half an hour before bed.

It is good to breathe slowly through your mouth with your tongue behind the upper teeth.

It is good to give thanks every day and be happy you are alive.

It is good to remember that people need and love you.

It is good to know you did your best, and leave the rest to God.

9 Health Tips

1. Drink unsweetened soymilk before bed. Soymilk will help you lose weight and it's good for circulation.
2. Eat 1-2 eggs every morning. It is best if the eggs are only 70% cooked. Eggs have high-density lipoprotein that cleanse your blood of cholesterol and supply you with adequate protein.
3. Eat more fruits than veggies. Always choose the most colourful fresh fruits and vegetables.
4. Drink green tea. Green tea is good for your brain as it protects the nerves. It can even help clear up skin problems.
5. Drink a cup of coffee every day. You can have coffee before you exercise. Do not drink coffee three months before becoming pregnant. Drink fresh ground coffee, as this is better for your health.
6. Eat yams at least once a week. They help with cell growth and prevent cancer. Yams are also good for losing weight. Red, sweet yams are the best, and bake instead of boil.
7. Eat steamed clam meat, as it protects your liver.
8. Do not microwave food, as it takes away some of the nutrients.
9. To stay slim: use less oil, less salt, less sugar, get more exercise, eat less but more often, and drink more water.

The Problem with Cold Drinks

It is nice to have a cold drink after a meal. However, the cold water will solidify the oily stuff that you have just consumed. It will slow down the digestion. Once this 'sludge' reacts with the stomach acid, it will break down and be absorbed by the intestines faster than the solid food. It will line the intestine. Very soon, this will turn into fats and lead to cancer. It is best to drink hot soup or warm water after a meal.

Jokes (Laughing is Good for You)

The Old Woman & The Lamp – An old woman found a magic lamp. The magic lamp became an angel and said to her, "You can make three wishes and they will come true." The old woman said, "I want to be beautiful, and I want to be rich, and I want my cat to turn into a Handsome Prince." The angel granted her wishes. The old woman became a beautiful lady with a lot of money, and a Handsome Prince appeared by her side. The woman was feeling very sweet and moved closer to the Handsome Prince, who softly said to her, "You made me so we cannot have sex. Are you happy now?"

Dead for the First Time – An old man passed away and his family had his body frozen. The day of the man's funeral was very hot indeed, and when the family removed him from the freezer, his body began to sweat. The man's grandson saw this and in a frightened voice said, "Grandma! Grandpa is sweating!" Grandma answered, "Well, this is the first time your Grandfather has died. He's just excited!"

Scariest Book Ever – June asked her father, "Dad, did you ever read any scary books?" June's father answered, "Of course I did! There's a book I've been reading for the past

58

20 years, and it scares me every single day." June replied, "Really?! Tell me, what is this book?" June's father, looking rather serious, replied, "The marriage certificate."

Sex Nowadays

Sex can be beautiful, but it can also be terrible.

Sex can be sweet, but it can make you cry.

Sex can be very challenging, even if you are very talented.

Sex can use up all your energy if you don't know how to control it.

Sex can make you feel high, so you can become addicted.

Sex can make you sick if you are not careful.

Sex can help you sleep, but it can also give you insomnia.

Sex is so good that you never have enough.

Sex never lasts and is never the same.

You might have enough sex, but I might need more (or the other way around).

You make love, but it doesn't mean you have to *fall* in love.

You can standby 24 hours ready for sex, if you find the right partner.

You might not feel like having sex, so you don't have to.

Men's Sexual Concerns
& Book 3

In June's third book, she will deal with the following statements and concerns, and much more:

1. I don't think my wife feels anything when I make love to her.
2. I notice my wife is very dry when we have sex and I lose interest.
3. I lost my sexual attraction to my wife after 10 years of marriage. What can I do to get it back?
4. I am a single father, and I lost my wife. I feel guilty when I touch other women. How can I feel better about sex again?
5. I am old now but I still have sexual needs. I want to be touched by women again, but I don't want to remarry. Can you help satisfy me?
6. I had my prostate removed and I lost my confidence and ability to respond sexually. My wife doesn't want to have sex with me anymore. What can I do?
7. I am inexperienced sexually and my girlfriend complains about my sex technique.
8. My girlfriend thinks my penis is too small. What can I do?
9. Sometimes my wife complains that I don't have enough sex drive. How can I boost my sex drive?

10. I ejaculate too quickly and I'd like to learn how to prolong sex.

11. I love sex so much, and I've masturbated every day since I was 13. I'm now 30 and I am not as sexually strong as I used to be.

12. My penis is overly-sensitive and I come too quickly.

13. I respond sexually only to my wife and not other women.

14. I only want to have sex with other women and not with my partner. Why?

15. Why do I have so many sexual dreams, but I am not a sexual maniac?

16. I can respond sexually only to fetishes, like my obsession with women's feet. I would like to be more balanced, and not need these fetishes to become aroused.

17. I can become aroused only when there is violence in sex. I feel bad about this. What can I do to understand myself better?

18. Why can't I come easily?

19. I need to be in love with someone before I can have sex with them. Why am I like this and others are not?

20. I am relaxed and comfortable only when I have sex with members of the same sex.

21. Why do I love to dress up as a woman when I have sex? I'm very much a man!

22. Why does my partner not want to have sex with me anymore?

23. I don't like to have sex with the same woman twice. I would like to understand why I'm like this.

24. I feel like I think about sex all the time, and I want to stop this.

25. How can I tell my partner that I don't want to have sex with her as often as she wants without hurting her?

26. I love to have sex, but my body doesn't respond.

27. I don't come as much as I used to. Why?

28. I don't come easily, but when I do it seems to be so much.

29. I love to be touched sexually, but I don't like to have intercourse.

30. My relationships don't last long because of sexual issues.

31. I don't like sex because I think it's wrong. I want to have a more healthy attitude about sex.

32. I have lots of sexual fantasies, but when I try them, I'm not interested anymore and I don't get as aroused as I thought I'd be.

33. Why do I always want to have sex with my partner's friends?

34. When I'm depressed, will sex make me happy?

35. Where can I find a good sexual partner?

36. How can I know if another person is sexy or not?

37. How can I have sex on a regular basis without losing energy?

38. How can I increase the amount of sperm I produce?

39. What are ways I can really arouse my partner?

40. I have decided to be a vegetarian. Will this make my sex drive better or worse?

41. I have a lot of sexual energy, and I get a lot of sex, but I'm still overwhelmed with all this energy. What can I do to balance it out?